Dancing in a THUNDER STORM

The Treatment and Care of the Alcoholic and Addicted Patients

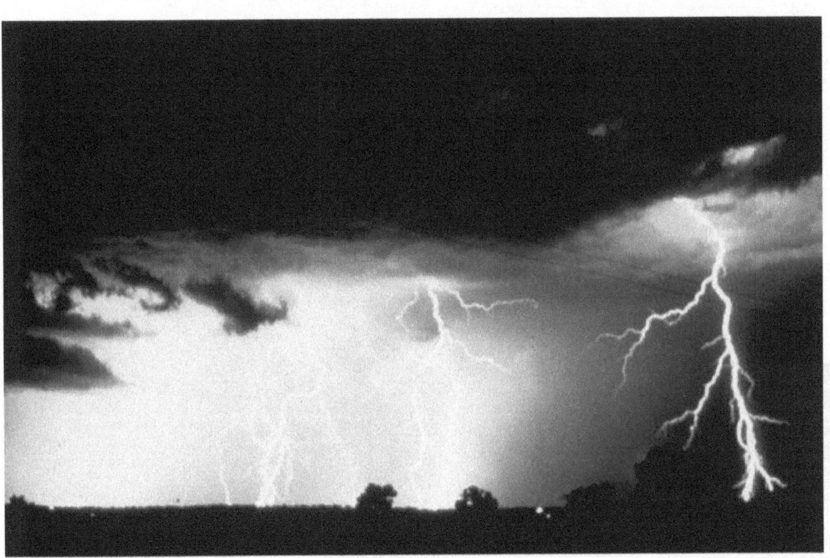

Edwin B Fuller

Dancing in a THUNDER STORM

The Treatment and Care of the Alcoholic and Addicted Patients

This is an Ozsolmon Book

Published by Edwin B Fuller

ISBN: 9781709995828

Chapter one: Introduction

Chapter two: Stopping the madness

Chapter three: What's the problem again?

Chapter four: Ok so this is what happened!

Chapter five: The restructuring of your life/ solving the reason you started

Chapter Six: Stories about recovery

Chapter One Introduction

Chapter One Introduction

The treatment of the addict is one of the most difficult things to do. There are many programs but it comes down to four things.
1 Stopping usage/ staying stopped
2 Recognizing the problem
3 Never forgetting the pain that it caused
4 The restructuring of your life/ solving the reason you started

All programs seem to have these four or five points. Like someone with one leg you will have to adjust to a new way of life, one that can and will support recovery. These Four parts to a treatment program are so difficult that in some cases it is impossible to fully help the patient. To make matters worse the treatment in its best form takes a long time. This can give room to disillusionment and frustration for the patient. This then causes mistakes and lack of focus which causes relapse.

One of the major things you are fighting against is the mind of the patient. In any painful event the mind tries to find a way back to normal. It tends to forget painful episodes and rewrite history. When a woman has a baby it may be the worst pain in her life but taken in context, the nine months of pregnancy, labor, and the beautiful child may seem more like a wonderful experience than just painful labor. This is what allows women to have more than one child. Childhoods, best friends and even accidents are rewritten by the brain.

This is a very important point especially for addicts. We often see the addict in pain and suffering. However the addict was also in a wonderful place with little or no pain were they felt great. The question is what they will remember. This is even more tragic for the alcoholic who has blackouts that mask his behavior and suffering from him. What he remembers is the wonderful drink not the driving under the influence or crazy argument.

The brain has played a trick on the patient and the patient is caught in a loop until the suffering has reached very serious stages. For this and a host of other problems the patient must stop using so a somewhat rational state of mind can exist. I mention this because often treatment begins and the patient is in acute distress and cannot rationally understand very much.

If the patient doesn't recognize the problem all bets are off. Unlike most other physical problems addiction needs the patient to get what is happening and accept there is a problem. Only then can the patient work against his own thoughts and ideas which will surely take him back to use.

Remembering pain or reality or an accurate history is so important that pains must be taken to get it correct. As the patient becomes better the reality will become clearer.

Lastly a complete life change is usually in order. What a user needs to have in order to stay clean and sober is structure. Lack of structure is the kiss of death because

there is a host of problems just waiting to surface. Addiction is a lifelong problem but with structure and awareness the problem can be arrested. In this step I have also added work on the cause. Once a person has gotten to this point it is important to return to the scene of the crime. Was it lack of structure, boredom, depression or the self-medication of a mental health problem that original allow the patient to use and abuse the alcohol or drug. The idea of dual diagnosis is very important. Another problem is often but not always mask but the problem of the drug or alcohol.
In some cases it is even more acceptable to have a drug or alcohol problem then a mental health problem. Cultural, sexual, ethnic differences can all have an effect on how the addicted is perceived and how the addict perceives themselves.

In the title of the book I used alcoholic and addicted to denote a type of difference in illegal and legal drug use and abuse and legal alcohol abuse. As crazy as it sounds many alcoholics are not doing anything illegal. It is perfectly legal to sit at home and drink yourself to death. On the other hand most drug abuse is illegal, even if the drug of choice is a legal drug. The reason this is very important is because the cultures in which the drug or alcohol is consumed. When I was in school studying alcohol abuse it was strongly stressed that alcohol is a drug. It is mostly regulated as a food product. Recent studies suggest that a small amount of alcohol or red wine may have some beneficial properties. Small amounts seem to be associated with a long life.

The cultural difference is very important in the treatment of the user. Alcohol is everywhere and is widely advertised and sold. Drugs are everywhere as well but require finding a dealer or committing an illegal act. Alcohol is cheaper by far than drugs which become more expensive as the user gains tolerance. These differences are very significant and may suggest very different approaches to treatment.

Lastly I would say that there are many very good books in the market place on this subject. The reason I have decided to write this book is because new approaches and treatments need to be developed for a problem that is so serious. In many ways few new treatments have been developed in the last 30 years but new drugs, attitudes about drugs (i.e. marijuana) and drinking patterns make development of new treatments more important than ever.

Chapter Two   Stopping the Madness

Chapter Two: Stop the madness

The idea that an addict or alcohol has to stop using in order to get help would almost seem obvious. The truth of the matter is it is very unclear how this is done.

Manually: Involuntary

Separating the user from the drug may be the hardest thing to do but manually doing it is very affective and if at all possible should be employed. The most common form of manual separation is jail. The user gets caught for a DWI and is incarcerated. After a time the user is rational and an intervention can occur. The longer the separation from drugs and alcohol the better the user will be. The user needs time for detoxification and healing. One of the reasons that jail doesn't work is because treatment is limited or nonexistent and the user usually returns to people places and things related to their usage. The fact that a person is separated from the drug doesn't mean they are clean. What it means is they are not using but even after years of separation the return to drug or alcohol use can be almost instantaneous when the person is no longer separated from his or her drug of choice. This phenomenon is called the dry drunk or dry use.

Sometimes users are caught by loved ones or professionals and detoxified in a locked unit or a private home or facility. This is probably illegal in the USA and several other countries. Unless the user is a minor or mentally unstable the user has rights. However this method if properly used it will bare very good results. The real problem with this method is nonprofessionals and loved ones who really don't understand treatment. If not done correctly this could back fire and send the user right back to the use of drugs or alcohol? It is hard to make someone hate something they love even if it is not good for them. *"The insanity of drug and alcohol addiction is not that people do crazy things when they are intoxicated, the insanity is that when they are sober they pick up a drug or a drink." Father Martin*

Voluntary:

The user will decide to stop using and go into a treatment program. This has several advantages over the manual approach. The user by his agreement to go to treatment is saying he needs help. Many things may happen but the user has at least said something is wrong. It is important to note that the user may not think the problem is drugs or alcohol. This is very common but it does give the counselor a starting point. In the treatment center the user will have peers and counselors and educational material. Treatment centers are great at education and therapy. The main drawback to this is that most treatment programs are too short (7 to 60 or 90 days, the standard is 28 days for 1st treatment) and they are for the most part voluntary and the user can quit and go back to using.

Long Term Treatment:

If short term treatments don't work the treatments that are long term may work. Long term treatments can be idea. The user at the end is normally very clear and rational. The user has been observed in various situations and has participated in a lot of education and therapy. Most 12 step groups recommend a year of sobriety before relationships or employment changes. The user has a program of recovery that has been used and evaluated. Most long term programs are from six months to three years with a year being an average. This type of program should have intensive after care and halfway house associated to them. If the user fails to stay sober then they can go back to the treatment and the failure could be a water shed experience and very beneficial for the user.

12 Steps:

Many users have stopped using by going to a twelve step meet. AA and NA and the two most popular groups that are for people who want to stop using. They are everywhere and easily accessible. This is the least restrictive way to stop using. Many users need more structure and it is not really easy to comprehend the principles. For must users they simply have to take the program on faith and do as they are told. These programs use sponsors, members who have been users but are now in recovery. This is somewhat hit or miss. A good sponsor can help the user to find his way but a not so good sponsor can frustrate and lose the new recruit. Most treatment programs introduce users to 12 steps and this is very helpful. However as I has stated before the is a well-tested method of recovery and millions of people with problems using alcohol and drug have gotten clean doing just A 12step program. Before Betty Ford and modern Treatment, 12 steps was the standard and it worked.

Different substances use different approaches to stopping. *Accelerated Neuro-Regulation (ANR)*
During Heroin detoxify using ANR or the Waismann Method sm, the body's opiate receptors are cleansed of opiates while the patient is anaesthetized and asleep. The goal is to rid the body of physical addiction: the patient literally sleeps through physical withdrawal. ANR eliminates the cravings that often accompany traditional opiate detox treatments.
The Waismann Method sm allows most patients to return to a productive life in a matter of days and eliminates the need to spend months in hospitals or rehab programs.
The Heroin detox treatment is performed in a full service hospital under the strict supervision of one of our medical directors. You are followed every step of the way from admission to release, and are assisted in creating a plan for remaining opiate-free once you complete your Heroin detox.
Waismann Method sm is proud to say that we have the highest success rate of any other Heroin detox facility. The Waismann Method sm allows most

patients to return to a productive life in a matter of days and eliminates the need to spend months in hospitals or rehab programs. the internet*

Heroin and opiates are often substituted by other drugs. Methadone, lamm, suboxone and subutex are just a few of the drugs used to replace the opiate. These drugs are also highly addictive but don't get the user high and allows for a somewhat normal existence. Normal is really in the eye of the beholder. Going to the methadone clinic every day to drink methadone is anything but normal.

Another approach to opiates is the use of Naltrexone®, so that if a patient should relapse, the drug would neutralize the effects of the heroin. This appears to work well but the user must take the pill every day and the user often stops coming so they can resume usage.

The essence of addiction

Stopping is a problem depending on how much you use and what you use. The phenomenon that separated drugs use from addiction is called tolerance. What tolerance means is that you need more of the drug to get the same effect the longer you use the drug.

Alcohol

One example would be that a college kid drinks a six pack once a week. In his second year he is drinking a six pack at least three times per week. In his third year he drops out of college and drinks every day. The next year he switches to vodka and drinks daily. In this example the progression is gradual but constant. For the alcoholic many times it is so gradual that the user doesn't realize what is happening only that he likes to drink.

Alcohol is a case of tolerance that happens slowly however it continues and appears to be inherited. The link is between father and son but may also include mothers and daughter. This is extremely important. There have been well documented cases where a person never drank and was brought up in a non-drinking household but when they finally did drink they drank alcoholically. This whole tolerance discussion would explain why certain culture can drink more than other cultures. The Irish have a high tolerance for drinking and cultural norms which discourage drunken behavior. In another case it seems that the American natives were not use to drinking and alcohol in a person with low tolerance is a recipe for disaster.

Tolerance then can explain binge drinking. There are people who only drink occasionally but every time they drink they drink alcoholically.

Drinking alcoholically is drinking far in excess of normal intoxication. This is made possible because of tolerance. In the party when everyone is saying man I'm buzzed and one person says not me, which is usually the person with tolerance. The person with tolerance loves the alcohol and can drink the normal drinker under the table. The problem with this type of drinking is that the body can't rid itself of this much alcohol so the poisons start to degrade the body. The liver, pancreas, and other organs are damaged. This also cases blackouts (the brain shuts down and the user doesn't remember what happened. Over time this can cause all kinds of problems including wet brain and even death.

Alcohol is in fact one of the most dangerous and damaging drug freely available to the population.

Drugs

The act of tolerance happens almost immediately with drugs. A user of heroin or crack cocaine will create tolerance with the first usage. This is one of the reasons that doctors are so careful about giving opiates to patients. These drugs are very strong and are good as masking pain but without proper supervision addiction can occur fairly rapidly.

In the case of cocaine and its higher potency brother crack the tolerance starts immediately and becoming addicted is almost immediate. This is the reason that crack addicts can spend every bit of money they have using drugs with devastating results. This type of drug produces paranoid thoughts. This results in a person in a corner doing the drug alone and in the end being so fearful that they don't answer the door, talk to friends or act rational. This drug also frequently causes cardiac arrest. The heart races and irregular heartbeats cause a heart attack.

Other drugs are very similar, valium, meth, and a variety of other drugs. Tolerance causes the addiction. Stopping only arrests the progress but the tolerance remains. This means that an alcoholic who stops drinking for ten years will drink alcoholically if they decide to start drinking again.
The use of drugs to stop

To stop a user from continued use psychotropic drugs have been used with some success. The use of LSD and other drugs have been tried and seemed to work but to my knowledge work was halted in the early sixties.
Drugs that help with depression or change thinking in a dramatic way could be useful. However these methods have not and are not widely used.

Hypnosis

Hypnosis has long been used to overcome some of the symptoms of addiction. It seems that different scripts address different subjects that may or may not be important to the user. Here is a script that focuses on the symptoms of withdrawal.

"Now as you go deeper and deeper relaxed, deeper and deeper on down, in your mind's eye, I want you to imagine the symptoms of withdrawal. I want you to feel the nausea. Feel your stomach turning. Feel all your muscles tighten.
Like you're tied up in knots and you feel terrible all over and I want you to take those feelings, take those feelings and you're going to associate them with the drug itself. You associate those feelings which represent the withdrawal symptoms with the drug itself, with the heroin or whatever you retaking.
From now on instead of the withdrawing causing the symptoms, the drug itself will bring the symptoms about. For your conditioned just as much as if I'd said a nice thick juicy steak smothered in mushrooms or if I asked you to concentrate on a lemon, you'd feel the saliva, the organs would respond, and now I say that the organs respond to the drug heroin or whatever you're taking.
The organs respond by producing very uncomfortable symptoms so from now on whenever you take a fix these very uncomfortable symptoms begin to show themselves.
As they show themselves, you feel them, you feel them deeply, very deeply. They are very uncomfortable. On the count of three as you withdraw from the heroin, the symptoms, instead of getting worse, get better. You feel better. More alert. More awake, more vital, more full of life. More full of

pep and energy than you have had for a very long time. You feel as though you are full of vitamins.
It's going to be very easy for you to withdraw because the withdrawing makes you feel good, and the taking of the drug makes you feel bad. You're going to be surprised about the reverse effect, but it's becoming a permanent part of your subconscious mind, never to be removed. Your need for heroin is gone. But you have a tremendous need to withdraw for if you don't then you feel the symptoms.
Now starting right at this moment, you're going to begin a new phase of withdrawal. A withdrawal without pain, without nausea, without vomiting, and without troubles.
Now I want you to feel good all the time, and the drug is the thing that makes you feel bad. The thing that gives you the nausea and the problems is the thing that ties up your guts, that's heroin.
Now as you go deeper and deeper relaxed, and as all of the sounds fade away in the distance, all of these suggestions take complete and thorough effect upon your mind, body, and spirit. And you sink deeper and deeper and deeper.
Nothing disturbs you. For you've begun your withdrawal right now. Now, sleep deeply and let these suggestions seal themselves in the deepest part of the subconscious mind. Way down."

I have read several scripts related to stop drinking and stop drug use however they seemed to be very badly written. For one thing in order for hypnosis to be worthwhile you must know the user. What are the user's fears and reason for use? Secondly you must know the disease of addict. It is not coffee is bad and you no longer want to do that.

The difference between Men and Women

There may not be that much of a difference between the sexes but there are some. Financing the drug use is one were women often use more, use longer and are more damaged by the drug usage. Women typically often start usage with a man, where he subsidizes her usage. The women can often get men to support her usage and may move into prostitution. Women tend to neglect their children and the children typically get removed from the home. There is an associated shame for women who are user and don't take care of themselves. Due to the wide use of benzo (valium and Librium) women often can be introduced to drug use by a doctor.

For men typical alcohol abuse then leads to all types of usage but the problem is that most men turn to crime as a way to support their usage. This typically means there are a criminal interventions, jail time and arrest associated with their usage.

This is simply a side note to say marijuana has been a gate way drug for many people but probably poses less of a threat to the community as a whole than alcohol. Medical marijuana and legalization of marijuana seems to be the future of the drug which may be good for society as a whole.

Chapter Three: What's the Problem Again?

Chapter Three: What's the Problem Again?

"Officer I just had two beers! It was my birthday and my friends made me drink, really I don't have a problem with drinking!"

You Honor, I've been under a lot of stress, I just had a new child and I've been working overtime and after work I went to the office party.

Get off my back honey, I work like a dog and you're always nagging me about something, If you would just clean this dump up I wouldn't have to drink!

I only drink once a year and every time these cops catch me!

If I don't use a little something I'll fall asleep, I work at night and I don't want to lose my job.

My back really hurts and the doctor stopped giving me the pills so I buy them on the street, it is just because of my back.

OK, OK, so I smoke a little weed, I'm so bored and depressed and the clinic won't refill my pills.

My friend has been shooting drugs for years and he doesn't have a problem, I think the dope has just gotten bad, I hope some better shit hits the street so.

All of the statements are not the problem but the user really thinks they are the problem. Denial and non - believe is the single biggest hurtle to overcome with a user. The drug or alcohol consumption is the problem and until the user believes it is the problem it will continue to be a problem.

Denial is simply the minds way of saying "I'm alright". Denial is a very important thing. When friends say why are you applying to Harvard? You will never get in. You apply anyway and get in. What a great feeling knowing you were right and your friends they were miss-informed or just jealous. In his way denial is important to ones sense of self and ego development. The major point is that the same thing that may have served the user very well in the past will betray the user once alcohol or drug use becomes habitual. The drugs and alcohol do all the work.

The alcoholic or drug user doesn't like the drug or alcohol they love it. It makes them feel great and as time goes on like anything people like the user will try to do it more and more. Other people often people close to the user see this and often confront the user but denial keeps the user on his path of usage. What separates alcohol and drug usage from say Pepsin or a chocolate addiction is tolerance. Tolerance is the secret weapon of drugs and alcohol. Tolerance simply means you need more of the drug to get the same effect. In alcohol it acts slowly and in drugs it acts almost immediately. In either case the user then increase his use of the product to get the same effect and in the process starts the damage to his mind and body.

Unless the user can identify and accept that they have a problem then as soon as they have free will the mind and possible the body will betray their wish to change and stop usage. Literally the user is dancing in a thunder storm and doesn't plan to get hit with lighting but the longer he dances the more the users exposes themselves to the lighting.

I actually know a man who has drunk himself out of a job and has alienated his wife and every time he drives he is very close to having an accident. He has been drinking for years and years and years. He always ask so gray question. So Ed what can I do? Thousands of times I have said stop drinking but not only has he not stopped in many cases he has increased his drinking. To hear him tell the story he is this wonderful man who has worked hard and been a great husband but this is so far from the truth that to people from the outside he seems crazy. The police have been called several times due to domestic disputes. This man was so intoxicated he could not work or care for his aging father. He cannot control his drinking and got fired because of it. However when you have even a brief conversation with this man the problem is his wife and the messy house. He has to drink in order to live in this situation. He can't move out because he loves her and yet he complains about her at every opportunity.

Why can't this man understand that he has a problem and get help? This is a forest for the trees problem but the real manager is the addicted brain.

This man has few friends and picked a woman who at the best would put up with his drinking, someone who is handicap. Next he found employment were his drinking went unnoticed for years. This is what I would call an envelope of addiction. Everything is a neat package of excuses and flawed logic that supports his assertion that he has to drink.

For the user like a bird he builds a nest for his need to use. The longer he uses the better the nest gets. The nest is usually very well put together and very hard to penetrate by time the user has problems with his using.

The envelope of addiction is what eventually kills the user. He can't switch gears or change and is living in an entrenched fantasy that is being controlled by his drug of choice. If you can stop the user from using but can't destroy the envelope of addiction then all is lost. This is one of the reasons that drug and alcohol treatment is so adversarial. Confrontation is needed to at least get the user to think in a new way.

One of the great ways that ongoing confrontation can take place is the therapeutic community. In a climate of treatment the peer have to talk about each other in terms of being truthful and honest and thinking correctly about what is really happening to them as a result of use. This is something that is really helpful in two ways. It is really easy to see the lack of rational and crazy thinking in others. One addict can really see how another addict can be lying or hiding from the truth. When you can recognize something in others it is much easier to recognize it in yourself. A user maybe able to outsmart a counselor but a group with clearly health group members will find the users weakness. This is because newly sober people who see the light are somewhat zealous about carrying the word. For these people recovery is a spiritual experience and a source of salvation.

In general you want this response because in time it wears off. As it wears off the newly converted former user will learn how to live without drugs or alcohol.

The problem seems like such an obvious issue. How does the user not realize this is the problem one might ask? The envelope of addiction doesn't seem to quit answer the question however the users don't see themselves as others see them. This issue will be discussed later in this book but for now I would like to say that the relationship between user and drugs or alcohol is an emotional one. The user has fallen in love with the drug or alcohol experience and it is not until the late stages of this disease that the user starts to have problems with the drug.

The AMA has given the addict/alcoholic a disease designation and this is true. Addiction/alcoholism is however one of the few disease that needs the user to participant in the arresting of the disease process.

Free Will

One of the major concepts in American life is the idea of free will. This is a great concept but it has some problems. Now let's start with an example. There is a seat belt law and if you are caught with it unfastened it will cost you $50.00. Of course this is free will, you can fasten the belt or not. Thinking about this law it occurred to me that if I rode a motorcycle which is far more dangerous than a car I would not have to wear a seat belt. The reason is it would be stupid. The real questions for wearing a seat belt is how many tickets ($50.00) you can afford to pay. This is an example of a negative consequence to a behavior. What if that negative consequence is death or jail? Free will still applies in most cases. The drunk who kills six people in a blackout still had free will when he decided to drink. He knew this could be a possibility or he should have known not to do it.

I work on a psychiatric floor at a major hospital and a man who tried to kill himself came to the unit and decided he wanted to leave but he could not because he had voluntarily signed in. He wanted to leave because he had something to do. Of course earlier he had tried to kill himself. What he couldn't understand is why he had to stay. This is another example of the lack of free will. The truth of the matter is any Doctor who let a man leave after a man came in an ambulance for an attempted suicide would be sued or loses his license and some more stuff. You do not have the right to kill yourself. The truth is if you succeed it is a moot point.

Now Patty Heist was also responding to negative consequences when she was in a closet and repeatedly stuck with sticks until she said what other people wanted her to say. This of course is called brainwashing and is not considered free will. The difference between Seat beat tickets and brainwashing is a grand canyon of gray. But I have come up with a formula.   Pain is a scale from 1 to 10.

The formula is Behavior times P (1-10) Consequences with no free will being P (> 8). Now freedom is Behavior P (<3).
Going back to the seat belt law in you had funds and could easily afford the fine then P (0). What makes P 0 is money.
The true formula for freedom is Money times P (0) times behavior X. I'm sure this is very crude but the fact remains if you can afford it then you are free to do it.

Using the same example if you crash and are hurt or killed the P (> 10) money not withstanding you are no longer free but at the will of your injuries. Some would say not wearing a seat belt, alcohol use, drug use and other dangerous behaviors are a threat to your freedom and free will. Also it show be pointed out that mental illness, health concerns and poverty all impede free will. So once again I must modify the formula.

P (< 4) + Money (x) + X behavior –the impeding forces of evil = Freedom = Free will

The problem with addiction and free will is that the user is always free to decline treatment. The pain scale is from other things other than drugs and alcohol. The police, my wife and my family, and just bad luck are the real problems that the user believes are the problem.

Unlike the case of Patty Heist we can't brainwash the user into sobriety. Many users have to me that they feel that treatment is brainwashing but unless the users can see the need for treatment or accept treatment then the user is at the risk of returning to use

Chapter Four: OK! This is what happened!

Chapter Four: OK! This is what happened!

Jack: I happen to have a drinking problem but I'm getting treatment for it and I've been sober for 6 months. I live with my wife and children who I didn't hurt because I mostly drank in bars and I plan to go home to them after this incarceration.

The reality is that drinking has finally upset the wife to the point where she is filing for divorce. The house is in foreclosure. His children are embarrassed and fearful of their father and have moved in with the mother's sister. The children had to change schools and are not really welcomed by the mother's sister and they blame this situation on their father's behavior. While incarcerated Jack has been fired. Even though Jack states he has been sober, he has had major urges to drink while incarcerated and he has hidden the fact that he has a stash of alcohol in the trunk of his car.

Unless the user can remember his pain he is doomed to make the same mistakes again. The crazy thing about addicts is not that users use. The crazy thing is that after they have not used and can identify how bad the drugs and alcohol have been to them that they return to using.

Some would say that Jack is simply minimizing his situation and that that is a form of denial. This may in fact be true but on some level Jack has re-written the history of his life. This is a more profound problem.

I once had a client who bragged about having a relationship with a really beautiful woman. Another member of the group came to me and said he knew the client and he must be crazy because he knew the girl he was talking about and she was anything but beautiful. I was confused by this and suggested that the girl had changed but the other member stated at the time the girl was homeless, smelled bad and was having sex to support a drug habit. I wondered how the client could have made such a great mistake. I asked the client to give a time line of his life and his interrelationship with this girl. It turn out that my client had seen this girl almost exclusively under the influence and his memory of her was tainted but his usage.

The client didn't believe me or the other client so we set up a field trip to see the girl and when he saw her he was astounded and started to cry. He attempted to talk to her but she didn't really recognize him and again he simply could not understand how he could have been so wrong.

The mind is a wonderful organ and it records what it sees as the client sees it. Also the mind can rewrite history to fit their view of how they see themselves. Lastly the mind collapses history often in a way that supports an overall view rather than a specific event.
The woman was in labor for 10 hours but was with child for nine months and a wonderful child was born. What the mind remembers is how she was treated by friends and family and a wonderful child. In the course of thing the ten hours of labor might not seem so big and she

thinking of it in that context may decide to have another child. Other women may decide to never have another child because not only was the labor bad but surround events were not good either.

Once I had a client who told me a very disturbing story. He had about a year and a half clean time. Six months had been in rehab and the rest in a halfway house. He had talked with his mother almost every week during this time but never went to see her on the advice from his sponsor. It was Christmas and he was invited to a family diner. He decided to go but he brought his sponsor just to insure nothing went wrong. His mother assured him there would be no drinking and the sibling were told not to drink and it was clear he would not stay very long. The meal went great but for desert the mother offers him cake which he declined. She was very insistent that he take some with him. Once in the car the sponsor said that something was wrong but he wasn't sure what it was. Half way home the sponsor stopped the car and looked in the doggy bag only to find that desert was a rum cake.

How could a loving mother make such a terrible mistake? The mother didn't think alcoholic she thought this was his favorite cake. Just because you change, the world doesn't always change with you. The rain on your parade is from people who love you, hate you or you are just in their way. The wicked witch and the flying monkeys are trying to make sure you don't get to OZ, see the wizard or go home. What most of the people in your world want is for you not to upset their world view.

Chapter Five: The restructuring of your life/ solving the reason you started

Chapter Five: The restructuring of your life/ solving the reason you started

Change is one of the hardest things anyone does. Moving, making friends, getting a new job, finding a doctor and keeping up with a new schedule would be hard for anyone but for the addict it is even harder. For most users the drug or alcohol was a crutch in most circumstances. The alcohol and drugs also stops the natural maturational process. If you started drinking at 17 then at 36 you will probably still have some teenage relate problems, like relating to the opposite sex.

OK the user stops drinking. What does he do now? In Jacks case he is a man with time on his hands. No job, no wife no children and bills and debt that are continuing to grow. Most professional would say forget life and focus on recovery. This seems to be a good plan because without recovery firmly in place nothing can happen. The first bump in the road and the user is back to using and no matter what he or she did it is all in vein. For most users the focus must be all encompassing and should become a restructuring of a life to fit recovery.

The key to restructuring a life is structure, structure and still more structure. Time, boredom, unplanned activities are all bad things. For most users these times represent their past life as a user. The people places and things often trigger memories of use in some former life far far away. The Idea is to have the user identify the triggers and do the next best thing. Triggers need to be talked about, explored and exposed. A trigger is a false representation of former usage which makes the former user wants to use again. This is a trick that the mind is playing on the user. Remember the fun you had when you were high but it fails to include the consequences of that usage. The user must think it through and Play the entire tape. The memory of pleasure must be pair with the consequences of that action. This is one of the reasons that AA and NA meets are so important. Many users actually don't like the meets because they remind them of the consequences of using but this is a good thing in that it help the pairing to take place and helps the user to remember the pain.

Structure will come to include employment which has to be sober friendly. When all your co-workers know that you cannot use and they don't use the environment becomes a safe place to work. Usually former employment is not a good idea. It really didn't support the user in the past and will probably fail to do so in the future. There are some types of employment that stand out as being inappropriate. One is any job that is done alone but provides cash and access to drugs and/or alcohol. Examples of this would be work in a bar, a taxi cab driver or a waiter. Other jobs may include high stress employment that requires special image control, lawyers, nurses and police. There is a problem when a former alcohol user arrest a DWI suspect. The arrest might go fine but the mind is now producing triggers that the former user is unaware of. It simply is not worth the risk.

Structure will come to include relationships, family and friends and romantic encounters. AA suggests that there should be no romantic encounters for at least a year. This is a very good rule. Learn to live and love yourself before taking you show on the road. Friends and family on the other hand may be a more painful problem. Who are the friends that support your recovery? There may be none. The fact is that most users upset many friends and family members. Move on in the early stages of recovery, later a user can try and make Amends. It is important to remember old friends and family may be of no help at all especially if their view of you is as a user. It is never surprising that friends and family may treat the user badly even if he is doing well because of built up anger over past behavior.

Solving the reason you started

Sometimes there is a question about why did A user start in the first place. To many counselor and health care professional this is a red herring. The chance to blame someone or something for the condition the user is now in. Many people will say that it doesn't matter why you started only that you stop and are able to stay stopped. This may be a very simplistic approach to what may be a very complex problem.

I believe it is true that most users started as a form of recreation or fun. If you are bored on a Saturday night what do you do? Go drinking with friends and hang out. Drinking then goes hand and hand with fun and free time. This may be as social as apple pie but for some it is the kiss of death. In recovery a good deal of attention needs to be placed on down time. The user must develop ways to stay active and develop new behavior for feeling bored.

I actually heard a very disturbing story about a school teacher who fell and hurt her back. She was on some pain meds but didn't think they were working well. She decided to increase the dosage on her own and by and by she started to go to multiple doctors and finally started writing her own prescriptions. Three years later she had lost her house her job and was living in a shelter and begging on the street.

She finally was accepted into a methadone maintenance clinic and her pain as well as her drug habit was under control.   Friends reported that although they did not believe she used again she was never the same. The drug experience had destroyed a wonderful person, her sister said. She no longer attended church, taught or socialized with friends and family. A relative that almost didn't recognize her saw her working at a fast food restaurant. She reported that her relative refused help and was difficult to talk to. The relative did not give up and made it a point to see her and take her clothes and some other items. Finally the former school teacher admitted that she lived in a shelter and was on methadone and was so ashamed of her situation that she really didn't want to socialize. This is not that uncommon that user who are no longer using are very fragile and are very focused on the here and now, take life one day, sometimes one hour at a time.

Peer or family pressure is another reason people drink. In many cultures drinking is part of the social network. In some cultures people drink with meals, ingest drugs on special occasions or use the drugs in a religious ceremony.   In the early sixties and seventies experimenting with drugs to get clarity, find nirvana and for fun was a certain type of norm. Some people simply didn't make it back from the trip that they were on.

When a user stops using usually there is a hole in their soul. There is good evidence that the hole was there long before the use of drugs or alcohol started. It is the hole that has to be filled in order for the user to feel ok. The use of structure and a new life may simply be a distraction from the hole. This is ok. There is absolutely no reason to do major personality reconstruction in recovery. However you must have the user learn new behaviors to deal with it. This is a tricky compromise.

The user is a 40 year old man named john who has recently stopped drinking and is doing well in recovery. He started drinking at age 13 with what could be described as abandonment issues. His mother worked long hours and the father was not in the home. The mother would drink on the weekends and was of exhausted during the week. John who was fearful of being at home along found that drinking sort of took the edge off. His half-sister Mary who was older would have male friends over who would bring beer and drugs to the house. When John was 14 one of Mary's girlfriends got in bed with john naked encouraged him to drink and then sexually assaulted him.

A year into recovery John tells his sponsor that he has been having sex with prostitutes and feels ashamed of his self and really has a distain for women in general and says candidly that he hates his mother. Recently his mother died and his half-sister has come back into his life. He asked his sponsor would he go with him to the funeral.

The emotional problems that John has are extensive and could derail his recovery. The primary objective is to keep john sober and rational. Even if he wanted to he cannot change his past but must fight to develop into a man who has enough self-worth to possibly have a girlfriend or partner and be able to stay sober and be honest.

John has several things working in his favor. He has a sponsor, he realizes that he has a problem and can identify feelings. This is a good foundation on which to build. Feelings will not kill him returning to use might.

On the negative side his sister is not really good in that her presence brings back the memories of a past life where he was a user and was abused. Even if she is in recovery her role in his life could be a trigger and not that helpful.

Chapter Six: Stories about recovery

Chapter Six: Stories about recovery

The Story of The
Man and his Monkey

Once upon a time there was a man who had a monkey and he loved his monkey and he was a happy man. Because he was attentive to his monkey he made sure to take special care of this animal. He washed it cleaned it and most important of all he feed it. As time went by the monkey grew bigger and bigger and bigger. In time the man started to notice that not only was his monkey growing bigger but he was also getting a bit out of control,. The monkey would eat all the food and ransack the house and destroy the inside of the man's car. One day the man was telling his neighbor about his monkey and how he loved the monkey but the monkey had grown so big and so bad. The neighbor stated that he had the same problem but he had found a very workable solution. What is it asked the man? Come with me the neighbor said. And with that he took the man into his back yard and showed the man a little monkey swinging in a cage.

Why that's just a little monkey. Yes my friend you are right he is little now because he is behind those bars and with my special diet he's getting smaller every day.

Do you think this can work for my monkey? Oh yes the man said I'm sure it will work but you will have to build the cage out of strong materials and once he is caged he can never be let out again. The cage was finally built. The two men immediately caged the big bad monkey and started him on the special diet. The man was so happy his monkey was under control.

As time went by the monkey became smaller and smaller and smaller and he found that with the monkey cage there were other things he liked to. The man found that he had time for a new job a hobby and a girlfriend and life was good better than it had ever been.

One day while his girlfriend was visiting she saw the cage in the backyard and asked what is that cage used for? Oh! Said the man that is the cage for my monkey. Monkey she said? Yea I have a monkey in that cage but you might have to look really close to see him. Oh I see him now what a cute little monkey can we take him out and play with him. Oh no said the man when he was out before he had become ugly and that's why he is in the cage now. But he is so small and cute maybe he'll be alright with me here.

The man thought and thought and thought and decided that the monkey was just fine where it has but his girlfriend refused to believe that there was a problem but let it drop. However as time went by and the man was involved in all of his other activities he forgot about the monkey. He stopped the special diet and through diner scrapes to monkey. As he needed materials for the other projects in his life he would from time to time borrow the materials from the beautiful cage that he had built. After all, the monkey was so small and the cage was so strong.

It was a quiet Sunday afternoon with the sun shining, laughter in the air, as he and his girlfriend strolled into the back yard. What happen to the monkey's cage and were was the little monkey? Much to their dismay the little monkey was a full grown gorilla and it was on the rampage. It destroyed the house it destroyed the car and it seriously damaged the man and his girlfriend. It was almost a year before they could even get a temporary structure up to handle this animal. By chance the neighbor saw the man and asked him what happen you had the cage and the special diet. The man hung his head and looking at the ground he said in a wee voice I forgot.......

What is the point of this story? The cage is a recovery plan. The special diet is people places and things. The monkey is your addiction. Please, Please, Please don't forget..........

Your pain is your salvation
Life is not fair
Everything matters
Nothing is free

Give God a place to live in your heart

WINTER MADNESS
A Baltimore tale

Winter Madness
A Baltimore tale

It was December 23, 2003 and a smart cat named Leon was sleeping at his desk. It wasn't so much that he was tired but that he as depressed. You see Leon wasn't getting paid until December 31 and he didn't have a single gift. His gas and electric bill was due, his phone had been disconnected and the credit card was maxed out. In short Christmas didn't seem that much like Christmas to Leon.

The 42 year old counselor and sometimes truck driver was marking time at the Westside counseling center and methadone clinic trying to figure out how the nurse made twice his salary when he had twice her education. What a depressing thought. What made matters worst was the fact that to make extra money he was also the urine monitor. Watching the vast array of penises sported by methadone addicts who often came in higher than a Georgia peacock on the CBS bill board simply made Leon sick. A violation of his own ethical stand of abstinence and greater stability through spiritual grow, methadone seemed a way to placate the addict while never addressing the addictive life style. Leon also believed that the move to methadone was a quick fix that was meant for black people and represented a racist approach to problem solving a very serious problem.

Leon, however his point of view would be changing nothing. It was too hard, too involved and definitely too much work. Besides he thought as he marched another client into the bathroom and looked toward the mirror what was the point.

As he glazed into the mirror something was wrong with this man's dick. How could a Blackman have a white man's dick?

"I'm sorry sir what are you doing? I won't accept this urine, Please go to the receptionist" he said in a calm but disturbed voice.

"Come on what's it to you?" as the client flashed a hundred dollar bill.

"It's nothing to me keep your money "! As Leon leaned against the wall he calmly said" Who are you fooling with that dick?"

"Nigga please what's it to you? And the client took of his watch and placed it on the stand with the 100.00 dollar bill. "Who will know?" Who will care?"

"I'll know and I care, come tomorrow without the fake dick and give a real urine. Besides I won't be here get the other guy but not me." With this the frustrated Leon went back to his desk to nap in his

misery. He closed his door and waited to see if any

more clients were approaching. Before he had barely

sat down there was a knock at the door.

Come in, Leon shouted but much to his

amazement there was the last client and his boss

standing in the door way. Dam what now? Leon was

sinking into his chair because a boss and a client

means trouble. There was the time that the client

claimed the Clorox came from the laundry he was

doing and of course the cold baby piss was because

the client had sleep outside all night. Excuses not

withstanding usually the client was given the benefit

of the doubt and life goes on. This of course erodes

the credibility of the counselor and enables and

reinforces drug addicted behavior. Leon was all too

aware that the boss was not interested in him but in the clinic.

As the two seem to stroll in as if nothing was the matter and the client was smiling Leon couldn't help but think that he was dead. What had he done and why was he in trouble? Leon braced himself, it didn't matter he thought he was not doing well and shit happens.

Leon this is Mr. James Mata from the department of parole and probation and no he is not a client.

Sorry but we had to know! I and my fake dick have been all over town and you were the only one to catch it and the only one to turn down the money and watch. We need integrity if we are to turn over the urine responsibilities to an agency. You guys have got the contract, congratulation. You should be proud but here is a little something for your troubles. In the envelope was five crisp one hundred dollar bills and a note saying Merry Christmas. Leon thanked the guy and thought to himself life is good!

A STORY ABOUT A STORY

Sometime the story is simple and neat and comes about because of an incident. As therapists with drug user sometimes the story help awaken abstract thinking which has not been used in that was in a long time. Mostly I have canned stories that are about changing behavior or managing sobriety. On this day however I had a group with women and this woman Anna who had used crack talk about how scared she was that she would relapse and would go back to drug use. I had told all my cool stories but I decided I wanted to develop a story to talk about her fear. However I was lazy and I decided to talk about the wizard of oz.

There was this cowardly lion and I think he over came his fear by talking loud and hanging with the right type of people and he found he did have

strength that he didn't realize he had. The wizard of oz

right Anna chimed in.

But that god dam lion hadn't been selling her

body and sucking dicks for the last three years for a

rock. I'm sorry Mr. Fuller I'm not even a lion.

I'm sorry Anna I'm just not on today maybe you

could tell me a story about how you will overcome

your fear and be successful in recovery.

Once upon a time there was a beautiful

women who was captured by an evil and mean

beast. She felt helpless and stupid because she went

willingly to the beast believing he was a princess and

would keep her safe but he did not. He beat her, hurt

her and treated her badly. Her mother had warned

her, her father had warned her and her girl friends had

warned her but she had ignored them all and gone to

the beast. The woman was so sad that she wanted to
die but the beast would not kill her or let her die. He
kept her alive to punish her for loving him and having
faith in him. He would taunt her for her mistake. The
woman lay awake at night wondering how she could
have made such a mistake. One night it came to her
that the beast was his most beastly self when he ate
from the zoom bush. She remembered that he had
always eaten from the zoom bush and that he
seemed to get magical powers from the zoom bush.
She remembered that she liked his power and beastly
nature when he ate from the zoom bush.

The woman now had a plan she would eat from
the zoom bush and as soon as the beast turned his
back she ate from the zoom bush and felt great. The
beast turned into a prince and made passionate love
to her and she was magically transported to a world

of pink and yellow flowers. In this place it was warn
and nice and she felt at one with her new
surroundings. When she woke up she thought she had
been dreaming was the beast a beast or a prince.
She must have been dreaming because the beast
was meaner than ever. She was in so much pain and
she had to run for her life. She felt terrible worse than
ever and the beast was angry.

With this Anna stated to Cry.

"Anna what the hell is the matter and
why are you crying", Jill stated in a loud somewhat
angry voice.

"Eat some Zoom and beat the beast's ass",
Mary joined in. "This story is sort of wacky if you catch
my drift. Why didn't you just leave the beast?

"Yea, it's like you want to blame everybody else
for what you didn't do.

By this time the group had run its course and I had to stop the group. Before I stopped I encouraged Anna to think of what her peers had said and come up with another story or an appropriate end for this one. I too was wondering how to help her see that she could stay sober by going to meetings and changing people places and things. I was really having a very difficult time thinking were I would go with this beast, zoom story. The next day Anna came to group with a big smile. She was happier than I think I'd ever seen her. Even some of the other patients noticed how chipper Anna was. As group started I said Anna you look pretty happy what's going on?

Well Mr. Fuller I've come up with a story.

OK let's hear it.

Once upon a time there was a girl who swam naked in a creek. It started to rain and she lost sight of land for a while and she became very afraid but the

she saw a bear drinking in the creek. She watched the

bear swim back to shore and thus found her way

back. She put on her damp clothes and the sun came

out the end.

"Wow" I said.

"Great job" Mary yelled and with that the group

started clapping.

The group went on to be one of the better

groups that the group had done and Anna remained

upbeat and positive during the whole group.

I never did see Anna again but the next day I

read an interesting article in the police blotter.

Apparently a circus bear had escaped and had

mauled a man badly near a local over run creek but

the police were interested in a woman seen at the

scene that was apparently swimming naked and

appeared to have been feeding the bear.

www.ingramcontent.com/pod-product-compliance
Lightning Source LLC
Chambersburg PA
CBHW051226250726
48655CB00006B/2613